TIME TO GET OLD?

Medical researchers have discovered that the body produces chemical signals instructing it to start shutting down—to slide into "old age" ... and that the hormone melatonin can block those signals! Besides its anti-aging effect, melatonin is also an outstandingly potent reliever of sleep disorders (including jet lag), and appears to be effective in stimulating the immune system and providing protection from many diseases, including cancer. In this concise guide to melatonin, the authors explain how it works, what it can do, and how to benefit from its properties.

ABOUT THE AUTHORS

Alan Lewis is a consultant to the natural pharmaceuticals industry, providing technical support services for many firms. With 15 years of study and activity in the field, he has authored numerous technical reports on nutritional medicine, nutritional pharmacology and metabolism, and is considered an authority in science-oriented nutraceuticals development.

Dallas Clouatre received his Ph.D. from the University of California at Berkeley in 1990, and pursues academic interest in philosophy, science and comparative medical systems. He has taught at U.C. Berkeley and the University of San Francisco. His book *Anti-Fat Nutrients* is in its second edition; he is also coauthor of the Good Health Guide *Diet and Health Benefits of HCA*. He acts as a consultant for vitamin and cosmetic companies in the United States and for herbal product manufacturers throughout Asia.

Melatonin and the Biological Clock

The amazing hormone that combats aging and renews health

Alan E. Lewis
and Dallas Clouatre, Ph.D.

Keats Publishing, Inc. New Canaan, Connecticut

MELATONIN AND THE BIOLOGICAL CLOCK

Copyright © 1996 by Alan E. Lewis and Dallas Clouatre

All Rights Reserved

No part of this book may be reproduced in any form without the written consent of the publisher.

ISBN: 0-87983-734-9

Printed in the United States of America

Keats Good Health Guides™ are published by
Keats Publishing, Inc.
27 Pine Street (Box 876)
New Canaan, Connecticut 06840-0876

Contents

INTRODUCTION

Melatonin was released into the general health and natural products market in the spring of 1993. This introduction, followed by massive consumer acceptance and enthusiasm, was attended by robust controversy in the industry. There were questions regarding its safety, the possibility of political repercussions and the appropriateness of the compound for sale in natural products stores.

The picture has changed. Several years have passed without negative incidents except for occasional individual reactions of a minor and idiosyncratic nature. Even before that, melatonin had a clearly documented clinical safety record over several decades (large or massive doses given to hundreds of subjects without harm). Now it is in use by hundreds of thousands of consumers, the vast majority of whom are very pleased with the product.

Further, there have been no political repercussions and the compound has gained general acceptance. Articles on melatonin either have been released or are about to be into the national media, and experts are already on the audiovisual media circuit. Melatonin is "hot."

Why this interest in melatonin? And do we have all the necessary answers?

MELATONIN'S POTENTIAL BENEFITS

Sleep

Melatonin's potential for improving the lives of users merits consideration if for no other reason than so many benefits have already been proven. It is a substance which is clearly an effective natural aid for encouraging relaxation and sleep. Melatonin thus addresses one of the most common complaints in contemporary society. Many of us are, after all, too often "stressed out." Melatonin is also effective in treating the condition known as delayed sleep phase syndrome and in correcting the disordered circadian rhythms of jet lag and shift work. Many pilots, stewardesses, business travelers, interns, nurses and others who because of travel and work keep irregular hours or hours "out of synch" with the sun swear by melatonin.

Immunity, cancer and aging

Melatonin is more than simply a natural "sleeping pill." There is an impressive and rapidly growing mass of literature on its ability to enhance the immune system. Researchers have studied the anticancer effects of melatonin, and melatonin appears to work closely with vitamin B-6 and zinc in opposing the immunologic decline which normally accompanies aging. There is good evidence for the antioxidant effects of melatonin and for the potential modification by melatonin of several neuropsychiatric, endocrine and metabolic dysfunctions which are typical of advancing years.

Mood

Though the literature on melatonin and neuropsychiatry is vast and inconclusive, melatonin may prove to be a useful adjunct in the treatment of some types of depression and other psychiatric disorders. A recent report described the use of melatonin to treat sleep disorders in hyperactive and neurologically compromised children: small nightly doses corrected the sleep problems, and researchers noted that improved mood and more stable and sociable dispositions tended to accompany the use of melatonin with these children.

Women's health

Melatonin has exciting potential roles in ameliorating women's health problems, such as osteoporosis, premenstrual syndrome, even birth control.

Melatonin clearly has numerous potential applications for health promotion and maintenance. As one of the body's primary anti-stress hormones, it performs what are referred to as tonic and adaptogenic functions.

CAUTIONS

In the usual sense of the term, melatonin is nontoxic. For most people even very large single doses, or multiple large doses given over several days or weeks, produce few or no side effects.

But remember that many of melatonin's actions are indirect: melatonin is a hormone which plays critical and not yet fully understood roles in regulating the production and secretion of other hormones in the body. The very nature of indirect effects can make it difficult for scientists to even recognize that there are connections, which is always the crucial first step to actually studying these interactions. *If there is a real weakness in our knowledge of the long-term effects of melatonin, it is in the area of this hormone's indirect influences on the body.* Fortunately, current research reveals that for many subjects, results previously obtained with melatonin in multimilligram doses can be achieved with 100s of micrograms instead. (To explain: 1 gram equals 1,000 milligrams; 1 millgram equals 1,000 micrograms; therefore 100 micrograms, for example, equals one tenth of a milligram.)

Modern air travel across time zones, the use of artificial lighting and the constant presence of electromagnetic radiation from many sources (the TV, the microwave oven, the clock by the head of the bed) all contribute to alterations in the rhythm of the pineal gland, which secretes melatonin. Therefore our everyday habits themselves can directly influence the natural production of melatonin. In many such cases the use of supplemental melatonin to correct what is already an artificial change in the body's cycles can have great benefits.

Nevertheless, caution is in order. The reader is urged to consider the section "Safety and Potential Side Effects" below which details these concerns, and to be aware that, except in microgram amounts, melatonin should probably not be used as an everyday supplement in the same way in which common vitamins and minerals are used. Reports are now appearing in the press regarding the antioxidant and free-radical-quenching properties of melatonin. But keep in mind that melatonin has other actions along with these antioxidant effects—the implications of which *for the long term* have not been elucidated.

Timing is critical

This point cannot be sufficiently stressed. Taking melatonin at the wrong time—opposing the normal daily cycle—can weaken rather than enhance immunity and is likely to have other untoward effects.

More is not necessarily better

You must find your (personal) optimal dose, which is the dose that has the desired effect without leaving you with a groggy feeling in the morning or any other side effects. If you can get the desired effect with less, *do so* (see the section "Finding Your Optimal Personal Dose" below).

Drug interactions and mood disorders

If you are using MAO inhibitors or other antidepressant drugs— that is, if you have a mood disorder—you should read the "Brain Function" section carefully and consider the implications in relation to your own condition before using melatonin. Unfortunately, the whole issue of melatonin in relation to mood (with collateral and significant connections to sleep physiology, hormone rhythms and the biological effects of light) is extremely complex and cannot be reduced to simple conclusions or prescriptions. Supplementary melatonin over time may help some and hurt others, or it may have no effect. If you elect to use melatonin, do so cautiously and observe yourself carefully; keep a mood log. If you are in serious doubt, refrain and/or consult with your physician.

Autoimmune problems

On account of the potential effect of melatonin on adrenal hormone levels (see the "The Pineal Gland and Immunity" section), and given that adrenal cortical hormones act as a physiological "brake" on autoimmune phenomena, these diseases are a red flag against unsupervised use of melatonin. Read the "Safety and Potential Side Effects" section carefully for more details and see the Appendix.

Pregnancy and lactation

The use of melatonin may influence other hormones sufficiently to be important in pregnancy, so caution dictates that it should not be used during pregnancy and possibly should not be used during lactation—certainly not without medical supervision. For more details, read carefully the sections "Of Special Interest to Women" and "Getting the Most From Melatonin: Dosage and Timing."

It should be noted again that melatonin is safe and without side effects for most people when used intermittently and in the proper doses as an aid to resynchronizing the body's internal clock—in case of jet lag or shift work, for instance. In other conditions, such as chronic insomnia, sustained use may be warranted. Melatonin is certainly a good alternative to current OTC sleep aids. It is best to experiment to find the lowest dose and frequency which yields benefit (see the section "Finding Your Optimal Personal Dose" below). Just as important, keep in mind that natural melatonin production in the body can be increased by techniques which produce sound and restful sleep (see the section "Increasing Your Body's Melatonin Production" below).

FINDING YOUR OPTIMAL PERSONAL DOSE

As mentioned above, more is not necessarily better. The watchwords are: *start low, go slow!* Given a choice, always use the lower dose.

Begin with commonly available 3 milligram (3,000 microgram) melatonin tablets, dividing each with a clean razor into 4 or 6 parts. Begin using these and watch for results. If results are not forthcoming, increase the dose until you find the level that suits you. Be sure to use melatonin only in the evening. You might also try using melatonin somewhat earlier than bedtime (say, around or after dinner: 5-8 PM). Some literature suggests that the optimal "window" for melatonin's clock-resetting effects varies more toward such an earlier time. Consider other lifestyle changes to alter your endogenous (internal) melatonin secretion: light exposure during the day, exercise in the morning and dietary carbohydrate at night (see the section on "Increasing Your Body's Melatonin Production").

The optimal dose can vary widely between individuals, apparently on account of drastic differences in the rate at which the liver metabolizes (destroys) melatonin. For example, one of the authors (DLC) happens to be extremely sensitive to melatonin, and doses in excess of about 0.5 milligram (500 micrograms) are too much for him. Meanwhile, the other author (AEL) finds that even doses of 10-20 milligrams have only a mild subjective effect on sleep latency (but marked effects on dream vividness and recall). This dramatic difference is reflected in the experiences of many of the authors' informal interviewees and to an extent in the literature now being published on melatonin as it becomes more popular and commonly available. Surely, there is much more to be learned about the physiology and metabolism of supplemental melatonin. Meanwhile, exercise appropriate caution while engaging in your own personal "clinical study" on its effects on *your* body.

Remember that melatonin regulates cyclic functions and other hormones in the body. A small amount can "prime the pump" and thereby initiate a change in metabolic cycles, such as the lowering of body temperature and inducing sleep. Further, small doses, over time, may compensate for the age-related decline in melatonin production, with derivative and desirable effects on age-related deterioration of body functions (see the section "Melatonin, the Anti-Aging Hormone?"). However, larger doses are not necessarily better, and there have been no very long-term studies to assess their influence.

For perspective, consider that the top researchers in the field do not agree on dose or even on the suitability of melatonin for nonprescription use. Russell Reiter, a leading academic melatonin researcher, takes about 1 milligram (1,000 micrograms) nightly and says "I've been taking it for years for jet lag. When we made the discovery about its antioxidant potential, I started taking it regularly" (*Vogue*, February 1995). Walter Pierpaoli, another academic researcher and author of a book on melatonin, uses 5 milligrams (5,000 micrograms) nightly himself and recommends doses ranging from 0.5 milligrams to 5 milligrams (mg) depending on the individual's age. On the cautionary side, Richard Wurtman, one of the earliest and most prolific academic authors on the subject, cautions against chronic ingestion of milligram amounts of the compound and against any nonprescription use.

As with most emergent issues in biology and medicine it will likely be some years—if ever—before the "top researchers" have it all sorted out sufficiently to come to a consensus. Meanwhile, the clear-cut acute and subacute (days or weeks) safety of even massive doses of melatonin ensures the safety of intermittent use of much smaller doses, with the possible exception of those in the special populations mentioned above under "Cautions."

WHAT IS MELATONIN?

Melatonin is a ubiquitous natural hormone-like compound produced by the pineal gland (embedded deeply in the brain) and by other tissues, for instance, in the gastrointestinal tissues. The hormone is involved in numerous aspects of biological and physiological regulation[1]. It sets and maintains the internal clocks governing the natural rhythms of body functions. Experimentally, melatonin modifies immunity, the stress response and some aspects of the aging process. Clinically, melatonin has been used in rhythm disturbances, sleep disorders and cancer. It possesses multifaceted and far-reaching biological effects.

A hormone is "a chemical substance, formed in one organ or part of the body and carried in the blood to another organ or part which it stimulates to functional activity" (Stedman's Medical Dictionary). There is nothing intrinsic to molecules of hormones that make them identifiable as such to an individual without prior awareness of the concept of hormonal activity. "Hormonal activity" is actually a much better expression than "hormone." Hormones are defined by their activity in the body, not necessarily by a particular chemical structure. In other words, "hormone" is as much a verb as it is a noun. But in deference to common usage, and for the sake of readability, here the word is used in its common sense as a noun. In spite of this, please keep in mind the problem with this usage.

The description of melatonin as a hormone is less than clear-cut for other reasons. Melatonin is synthesized in several tissues (not only in the pineal gland, which is one of the ductless glands of classic endocrinology)[2]. It occurs in a wide array of life forms, including unicellular organisms and plants (which obviously have no endocrine system or hormones in the classic sense). Finally, it does not necessarily act via membrane receptors—a phenomenon closely associated with definitive hormonal status in contemporary endocrinology[2]. This means that melatonin does not need to interact with a special receptor on the surface of cells in order to exert its effects.

Melatonin occurs in human milk[3] and in a variety of common plant foods[4] such as bananas, beets, cucumbers and tomatoes. The occurrence of melatonin in vegetation parallels the occurrence of its precursor compound serotonin, which has long been known to occur in plant materials, particularly tropical fruits. Animals given foods high in melatonin have demonstrably elevated levels of plasma melatonin[5], and researchers speculate that humans may likewise obtain biologically active quantities of melatonin from their diets.

We also consume the building blocks for melatonin in many foods which are noted for aiding sleep. One of these is cow's milk; the warm cup at bedtime supplies the amino acid tryptophan. Chemically, melatonin is N-acetyl-5-methoxyserotonin—a methylated and acetylated derivative of serotonin, which in turn is derived from tryptophan. One of the enzymes involved in this process is known by the rather formidable name hydroxyindole-O-methyltransferase (HIOMT). Serotonin undergoes several intermediate steps to form melatonin[6]. *The practical significance of the chemistry is that melatonin, in contrast to serotonin, is lipid-, that is, fat-soluble.* It readily crosses membranes and enters the brain and other tissues—even tissues without melatonin receptors.

Nightly melatonin levels depend not only on the foods eaten, and thus the amount of "building blocks" available, but also upon how active the person has been during the day. Some of the same hormones which activate the metabolism for a race around the block or for the thermogenic response to food need to have been activated during the day to improve melatonin production. More technically, melatonin synthesis depends upon cells remaining receptive to hormonal stimulation at "beta" receptors. This is called intact beta-adrenergic receptor function and it is stimulated by beta "agonists." Norepinephrine, the prototypical beta-agonist[7], activates the necessary step for melatonin production. Predictably, beta-receptor blockers, which are commonly given to lower high blood pressure and for other cardiovascular problems, depress melatonin secretion[8].

The enzymes of melatonin synthesis are activated and depressed, respectively, by darkness and light. The pineal gland, which is sometimes called the "third eye," receives light signals by nerve impulses. Release of melatonin follows a circadian rhythm: this simply means a day/night rhythm inasmuch as the word literally means "circa" (about) "dias" (a day). The circadian rhythm rises and falls in a 24-hour pattern that is to some extent controlled by light. The phases of light and darkness act as synchronizers of the pattern and determine the timing of the rise and fall[9]. Thus, during the night (or in darkness) pineal activity and melatonin synthesis and release are increased[7], and during the day (or upon exposure to bright light) they are depressed and sometimes barely measurable[6]. Melatonin has been described as the "hormone of darkness"[10].

The degree of rise and fall of melatonin (and other rhythmic hormones and processes) is referred to as amplitude: low valleys and high peaks make for high amplitude, while a flattened curve is of low amplitude. The significance of amplitude will become clear in the following sections.

Apart from being influenced by environmental light/dark cycles, the pineal, through melatonin, conditions the internal environment by setting and maintaining the internal clocks governing the natural rhythms of body function. This apparent clock-setting property of melatonin has led to the suggestion that it is a "chronobiotic" —a substance that alters and potentially normalizes biological rhythms. The influence of melatonin on biochemical and physiological processes is so broad that it seems unlikely that it works primarily by exerting direct effects. Rather, it appears that melatonin manages and adjusts the timing of other critical processes and biomolecules (hormones, neurotransmitters and so on), which in turn exert numerous peripheral actions[11].

BRAIN FUNCTION

Before the recent spate of scientific research, some physiologists had maintained that the pineal gland is vestigial, or without real function. However, no one now doubts that the pineal gland's secretions have real and significant roles in regulating brain function. Melatonin stabilizes the electrical activity of the central nervous system and causes rapid synchronization of the electrical activity of the brain as well.[7] In contrast, loss of the pineal gland predisposes animals to seizures. It has been proposed that the pineal, acting mostly but not exclusively through melatonin, is a "tranquilizing organ on behalf of homeostatic equilibrium," and that it "acts as a general synchronizing, stabilizing and moderating organ".[7] This suggests that melatonin may have many applications for stabilizing and harmonizing aspects of brain function and chemical production.

The relation of melatonin to depression has attracted great interest in psychiatry. Various forms of depression are related to disorders in the timing and the amplitude of the release of melatonin into the system. Nighttime melatonin levels are low in subjects with major depressive disorder and panic disorder [47, 48]. This is particularly marked in subjects with abnormal pituitary-adrenal responses to prescribed corticoids (synthetic adrenal hormones)[29] and who at the same time have disturbed corticoid secretion patterns. Normal individuals with mild or episodic depression also had lower than normal nocturnal melatonin levels[29], as did subjects with melancholic depression[49]. In contrast, higher than normal melatonin levels have been observed in manic subjects during the manic phase[49]. More significant than changes in the absolute amount of melatonin produced at night, the amplitude of the circadian melatonin rhythm is blunted in depression and becomes normal on recovery[50]. (See the discussion of circadian rhythm below.) *This means that in depression the ability to limit melatonin production discretely to the sleep period is typically not properly regulated.*

Human mood levels in general, not just in cases of disorders, reflect the pattern of release of melatonin from the pineal. Usually this pattern is influenced by changes in exposure to light. Good evidence suggests that the length of the day, the strength of light exposure, the timing of physical activity and similar elements influence the pineal gland and through it the release of melatonin and the individual's mood. The linkage of melatonin levels and pineal function with mood disorders is strengthened by epidemiologic evidence of human populations as this reflects the biological effects of light. Both Seasonal Affective Disorder (SAD, sometimes called "atypical depression") and classic "nonseasonal" depressions have a marked seasonal incidence with peaks in the fall and spring, respectively[51, 52]. This coincides with the troughs of the circannual melatonin rhythm[53]. HIOMT, one of the enzymes of melatonin synthesis, rises and falls in an annual rhythm, with troughs in March and October and peaks in January and July[54].

Clinical depression, unlike seasonal forms, seems to be partially unlinked to light exposure. The authors of seminal studies on melatonin in depression have proposed the existence of a "low melatonin syndrome" characterized by low nighttime levels of melatonin, disturbed rhythms of adrenal hormone release and *little* daily and annual cyclic variation in symptoms of depression[29]. Interestingly, depressed individuals who had lost a parent before the age of 17—an apparent conditioning factor for depression— had lower nocturnal melatonin amplitude levels than those who had no such loss[29]. This suggests that correctly timed melatonin supplementation may be an experimental treatment for depressed individuals with adolescent trauma.

Depression comes in many forms, but a common element may be an inability to properly respond to the body's hormones which are intended to stimulate activity. The best known of these hormones is adrenaline, the "fight or flight" hormone. Each cell of the body contains "receptors" designed to respond to activation signals (beta-receptors) and to turn off this response so as not to overtax the metabolism (alpha-receptors). The preceding section mentioned that activation of these beta-receptors during the day is required for the synthesis of melatonin. This fact provides a clue to one possible cause of depression.

The requirement of intact beta-receptor function for melatonin synthesis, and the stimulatory effect of norepinephrine on melatonin synthesis and release[7], point up a theoretic relation of melatonin to depression. A substantial body of evidence suggests that suboptimal activity of norepinephrine is involved in at least some forms of depression[55, 56] and it even has been proposed that depression is a "norepinephrine-deficiency disease." Antidepressant medications typically are designed to influence the amount of norepinephrine produced and/or the responsiveness of cells to this hormone. Many of the tricyclic antidepressants and all the monoamine oxidase (MAO) inhibitors enhance norepinephrine activity[57]. *The tricyclic antidepressant drugs dramatically increase melatonin synthesis in humans*[58]. Thus it is possible that the relation of norepinephrine action to affective disorders is mediated in part by effects on melatonin synthesis or on the amplitude of melatonin release. Tricyclic drugs often have sedative effects (melatonin enhancement?) and for this reason are often administered at night—an appropriate time for enhancement of melatonin rhythm amplitude.

Beta-receptor blockers, such as those used to control high blood pressure, depress melatonin production and secretion[8] and can alter the cycles of its production as well. They can also cause neuropsychiatric problems such as nightmares, insomnia, lassitude, dizziness, nighttime hallucinations and depression[59, 60]. When tested, those users of beta-receptor blockers who are plagued with nightmares and other sleep disorders have markedly lower melatonin levels than treated individuals without such symptoms[60]. Thus it seems that there is much individual variation in the sensitivity of the pineal to beta-blockers.

Brain serotonin levels are increased by melatonin administration[61], probably because some serotonin that otherwise would be required to produce melatonin is spared. This may be a significant finding since serotonin has been linked with an array of neuropsychiatric disorders. Much of the popularity of the now unavailable amino acid tryptophan was due to this compound's role as a building block for serotonin and therefore to improved serotonin levels in the body. Diminished serotonin levels in the central nervous system, as indicated by low levels of a serotonin marker in cerebrospinal fluid, are associated with impulsiveness, aggression and autoaggression[62-64]. Serotonin inadequacy may predispose individuals to many "disorders of constraint," including impulsive violence, alcoholism, compulsive gambling, overeating and other obsessive-compulsive behaviors[65, 66]. Support of the serotonin system with serotonergic nutrients or drugs can elevate mood, reduce aggression, increase the pain threshold[67], reduce anxiety[66], relieve insomnia[68], improve impulse control and ameliorate obsessive-compulsive syndromes[66]. By virtue of its effects on brain serotonin, melatonin might thus influence sleep, mood, eating, addictive and related disorders.

There have been no systematic studies on the potential of melatonin for use in the treatment of depression, but indirect evidence is suggestive. The drug psoralen, which exaggerates nocturnal melatonin release, has anti-depressant effects[69]. The potential of melatonin to treat depression will probably be realized, if it exists, as part of a multifaceted therapy involving properly timed bright light exposure and other techniques. Here are a few of the possibilities:

Seasonal Affective Disorder (SAD) is characterized by late sleep, overly deep morning sleep, increased appetite and retarded onset of nighttime melatonin release. SAD subjects appear to suffer from an abnormally delayed response to changes in light—technically, they are probably "phase-delayed" or "night people"[70,71]. SAD typically begins in the fall and persists through the winter[52]. SAD sufferers may benefit from induced phase advance (and light phase lengthening) effected by exposure to bright, pre-dawn light in the morning, early rising (to the point of sleep deprivation, for example, rising at 3-4 AM), and melatonin administration before bed, which should be early in the evening. High-dose vitamin B12 may also be useful for phase advance (see the section below on Complementary Nutrients). If naps are needed, it is important that they not be taken before midafternoon[72].

Classic endogenous or "nonseasonal" depression is characterized by insomnia (especially early morning awakening), appetite depression, weight loss and the advanced onset of nocturnal melatonin release. Those suffering from this form of depression may be "phase-advanced" "morning people," although not very effective ones[71]. Classic depression typically begins in the spring and persists through the summer[52]. This group might benefit from induced phase delay (and light phase shortening) effected by bright light exposure in the evening[70], later rising with avoidance of bright light in the morning and delayed-release melatonin in the late evening or immediately before bed.

A warning is in order. Melatonin administration which prolongs the nocturnal melatonin rise may exacerbate SAD[73] and bipolar and classic depression[74]. In one study, very large quantities of melatonin (1 gram/day) were given in divided doses through the day, thus abolishing the normal daily melatonin rhythm and increasing symptoms[50]. Melatonin should be used only with caution in depression (see section below titled "Safety and Potential Side Effects"). Its administration should always be appropriately timed and always be combined with light therapy and appropriate changes in sleep phase.

TO SLEEP, PERCHANCE TO DREAM: RESETTING YOUR INNER CLOCK

Melatonin is a useful aid in insomnia. Low-dose oral or nasal melatonin (from 0.1 to 10 mg) has significant hypnotic effects in normal humans. Experimental subjects given melatonin reported feelings of well-being and emotional balance after the sleep period. Melatonin also has anti-anxiety effects similar to popular drugs such as Valium.

Several lines of evidence suggest a relation among sleep, pineal function and melatonin levels. Nighttime melatonin levels and the quality of sleep both decline at puberty[12]. In the elderly, melatonin levels have declined dramatically from those of youth, and sleep tends to be both shorter and poorer. Of all the claimed benefits of melatonin, those of aiding sleep and resetting disturbed sleep patterns such as come with jet lag are the most solidly supported by research.

Trials have shown that melatonin corrects the sleep disturbances, mental inefficiency, and daytime fatigue cumulatively known as jet lag—the biological rhythm disorganization caused by the sudden change of environment and associated light/dark cues—that occurs after plane flights over several time zones[13,14]. However, *melatonin taken before travel can actually worsen symptoms, in contrast to the benefit of melatonin taken immediately upon arrival*[14]. *Good results are typically found by taking 1 to 3 mg melatonin from 1 to 3 hours before going to sleep in the new time zone.*

Supplemental melatonin has been used successfully in delayed sleep phase syndrome—a type of insomnia characterized by wakefulness past conventional bedtime and inability to fall asleep before 2-3 AM. Small doses (5 mg) of melatonin given at 10 PM resulted in advance of the sleep phase (shortening of time to sleep) by about 1.5 hours[15, 16]. In one of these studies melatonin was shown to reduce sleep duration by about 30 minutes[15], suggesting a decreased sleep requirement consequent on improved sleep quality.

The delayed sleep phase syndrome is considered an unusual (low-incidence) form of insomnia. However, it is possible that many "night people" —individuals who favor activity late into the evening or night, with a correspondingly slow start and feelings of malaise the next morning—are affected by a subtle variety of this phase-delayed condition. These individuals might wish to attempt an experimental lifestyle alteration with well-timed supplementary melatonin (see discussion of Seasonal Affective Disorder above).

Melatonin has also been used to alter sleep architecture in narcolepsy—a disorder of disturbed circadian sleep/wake rhythm and rapid eye movement (REM) sleep deficit where sufferers sleep poorly at night and fall asleep during the day. Changes in REM sleep patterns similar to those of narcolepsy also occur in animals and humans after removal of the pineal gland[17]. Pharmacologic doses of melatonin (50 mg) dramatically increase REM sleep time in both narcoleptics and normals and greatly intensify subjective dream phenomena[17].

Several studies have demonstrated the sedative and sleep-inducing effects of supplementary melatonin[7], although there is considerable inconsistency in reported side effects. In one study, high doses (80 mg) of melatonin given to healthy subjects were reported to exert "a hypnotic effect by accelerating sleep initiation, improving sleep maintenance and altering sleep architecture in a similar manner to anxiolytic sedatives; ... [the results] indicate good tolerance of one dose of melatonin without hangover problems on the following morning"[18]. Ultra high-dose melatonin (240 mg/day) caused sedation and slower reaction time without significantly impairing memory[19], which contrasts with a number of drugs, such as the benzodiazepines. Melatonin is reported to have anti-anxiety effects and (in vitro) benzodiazepine-like actions[19]. Low-dose (1.7 mg) melatonin given as a nasal spray at 9-10 AM induced sleep within 1 to 2 hours in 70 percent of recipients[20]. All subjects reported feelings of well-being and emotional balance after the sleep period.

Low-dose (2 mg) oral melatonin given at 5 PM can increase subjective sensations of fatigue[21]. This is followed the next morning by decreased fatigue, suggesting phase advance of a subjective energy rhythm and possibly improved sleep quality. Low doses of melatonin (range: 0.1 to 10 mg) given to healthy males have significant hypnotic effects relative to placebo[22].

In contrast to the lack of side effects reported in the study above using 80 mg per night, at least one student of melatonin who uses the hormone in his medical practice found that amounts above 6 mg seemed to routinely cause grogginess, "fuzzy thinking, and lethargic feeling" the next morning. More than 200 subjects were surveyed. Few side effects were reported at 3 mg and almost none at 1 mg or less[157]. With proper timing and forms of administration, it may be possible and preferable to use dosages of as little as 100 mcg to achieve melatonin's sleep-inducing effects.

Sleep-disordered breathing and snoring, characteristics of the sleep apnea syndrome, have recently been found to affect 9 percent of women and 24 percent of men in the general population[23]. Sleep-disordered breathing and sleep apnea are associated with daytime sleepiness and cardiovascular disease. It is possible that melatonin supplementation, by improving the quality of nighttime sleep, could play a role in the management of this very common and sometimes disabling condition.

Melatonin has been used successfully to treat serious sleep disorders in hyperactive and neurologically compromised children. Doses of 2.5 to 5 mg nightly were used with prompt sedation and improved sleep quality noted in almost all the (15) subjects. No side effects were reported. There were other benefits, as well: "Improved mood and disposition [of the melatonin-supplemented children] have been the rule. Irritability has been greatly decreased and age-inappropriate temper-tantrums have disappeared. The children have tended to become more alert and sociable, and developmental gains have often been noted"[24]. These findings are consistent with the postulated role of melatonin and zinc in attention-deficit hyperactivity disorder[25].

The stabilizing and synchronizing effect of melatonin on brain electrical activity was mentioned already. During periods of deep relaxation such as Transcendental Meditation, blood levels of pineal indoles are increased[7], and a recent study demonstrated increments in urinary melatonin metabolites (indicative of elevated blood melatonin levels) in subjects practicing "mindfulness meditation"[135]. Current research on the pineal and on melatonin has provided some preliminary support for the romantic conception of the pineal as "the morphological substrate of the seventh 'Chakra,' being the gateway to perfect rest and harmony"[7]. A combination of melatonin with vitamins and accessory factors may constitute a useful experimental tool for circadian rhythm synchronization, lucid dreaming (conscious control of the dream state and its content)[134], dream analysis, visualization and meditation.

Pharmacologic doses of melatonin (50 mg) dramatically increased REM (rapid eye movement) sleep time and dream activity in both narcoleptics and normals: "the narcoleptics reported intense colored dreams, completely devoid of their usual nightmare-like elements ... [normal subjects reported] dreams with intense colored visual imagery"[17]. Volunteers receiving high-dose melatonin (about 80 to 100 mg) experienced increased alpha brain wave activity and a feeling of well-being and elation which persisted for several hours [7,137]. Melatonin also increased REM sleep time and resulted in "abundant and vivid" dream episodes. Most recallable dreams occur during REM sleep, and REM sleep deprivation is characterized by anxiety, overeating, behavioral disturbances and decreased concentration and learning[138]. REM sleep seems to enhance memory and the resolution of emotional events. It is decreased in the mentally retarded[139]. Most REM sleep occurs in the two hours before awakening—the period of most vivid dreams.

Many psychotropic drugs, such as LSD and cocaine, increase melatonin synthesis[74]. It has been suggested that nonpolar (lipid-soluble) indolic hallucinogenic drugs (LSD) emulate melatonin activity in the awakened state[26] and that both act on the same areas of the brain[140]. While melatonin is clearly not a wake-state hallucinogen as is LSD, it may have mild effects during sleep. Melatonin chemically is 5-methoxy-N-acetyl-tryptamine, and tryptamines derived from native plants are known to induce hallucinatory experiences as used in some parts of South America by shamans[157].

The enhancement of the metabolism of vitamin B-6 (pyridoxine) by melatonin is discussed below. Supplementary pyridoxine (without melatonin) often enhances dream recall[141], and sustained-release pyridoxine preparations taken before bed may be especially effective (AEL's personal observation). Again, coadministration of riboflavin (vitamin B-2) is advisable since pyridoxine metabolism depends on this vitamin[117].

Dimethylaminoethanol (DMAE), a metabolic intermediate and precursor of choline, has been used to induce lucid dreaming[142]. This observation has some biological basis since DMAE is a cholinergic compound (fosters formation of acetylcholine) and cholinergic drugs increase REM sleep time[143].

Vitamin B-12 is reported anecdotally to intensify dream coloration, though high doses (1 mg) must be used and tolerance develops quickly[144]. High-dose vitamin B-12 (3-4 mg/day) has been used successfully in the treatment of rhythm disorders characterized by non-24-hour cycles of sleep and waking (for example, 25-hour "days")[145]. High-dose vitamin B-12 (3 mg/day) phase-advanced by over an hour the 24-hour melatonin rhythm in human volunteers and markedly increased their sensitivity to bright light-induced melatonin suppression[146], suggesting a role for the vitamin as an adjunct to bright light therapy of depression. However, the vitamin did not affect sleep/wake cycle rhythms. The combination of melatonin and vitamin B-12, along with morning bright light, would likely accentuate melatonin amplitude and phase-advance both melatonin and sleep/wake cycle rhythms, with implications for Seasonal Affective Disorder.

Pyroglutamic acid is an amino acid derivative that occurs naturally throughout the body and is present in many common foods[147,148]. It accumulates in the brain when administered orally and serves as a precursor of glutamic acid, an amino acid with cognition-enhancing properties. Pyroglutamate is structurally very similar to the piracetam family of cerebroactive, cognition-enhancing compounds ("nootropics"). Both pyroglutamate and glutamic acid serve as precursors of GABA, a sedative and antidepressant neurotransmitter that may have a role in circadian time-keeping[149]. Pyroglutamate enhances the release of acetylcholine, antagonizes drug- and shock-induced amnesia and partially corrects memory deficits in aged humans[150]. Glutamic acid has been suggested as a treatment for senile dementia (though pyroglutamate would be a better candidate). Pyroglutamate is also a precursor of glutamine, an amino acid with mild sedative and antidepressant properties, which may also enhance dream recall[151].

The optimal formula for rhythm synchronization, lucid dreaming and meditative activity might therefore include melatonin, pyridoxine, riboflavin, DMAE, vitamin B-12, pyroglutamic acid and perhaps glutamic acid or glutamine, to be taken in the evening or before bed. Sustained- or delayed-release technology will more closely mimic the natural nightly crest of melatonin and may help deliver pyridoxine and other factors to the brain during the pre-dawn REM/dream period.

THE PINEAL GLAND AND IMMUNITY

Melatonin reduces or modulates several harmful effects of the adrenal steroid hormones known as corticoids. These effects include
immune depression[30] and the excessive breakdown of tissues (lean
tissue wasting or hypercatabolism), or, conversely, weight gain,
shrinkage of the thymus gland (which produces the T-cells of the
immune system) and suppression of adrenal functions[31]. These
findings have led to the suggestion that melatonin "might be working
as an anti-adrenocortical or anti-stress factor in human physiology"[31].
The relation is reciprocal since nighttime stress or corticoid administration depresses pineal melatonin levels and likewise the levels of
the rate-limiting enzyme of melatonin synthesis[32].

There is a close reciprocal relation between the pineal and the
pituitary/adrenal axis. This special relationship between these two
glands controls body weight, blood pressure, stress response, immune function and other aspects of physiology. Melatonin modulates the activity of this axis as well as the actions of corticoids in
the body at large. Melatonin releases vasotocin, which lowers corticoid levels[26]. Removal of the pineal causes adrenal hypertrophy
(enlargement), which is reversed by melatonin administration, and
melatonin itself induces adrenal hypotrophy (reduction in size)[27].
There is controversy as to whether this represents a direct effect on
the adrenals, an inhibition of the release of corticotropin releasing
hormone (CRF), or other actions[7]. Effects on mechanisms of the
hypothalamus and pituitary glands constitute the most likely an-
swer since inhibition of adrenal function by melatonin does not
occur in animals with surgically altered hypothalamuses[7]. It has
been proposed that melatonin acts as a CRF-inhibiting factor and
thereby prevents damage to the immune system. In major depression, in which melatonin levels are low[28], the pituitary/adrenal
axis is overly active due to a lack of this modulating influence by
the pineal[29]. Melatonin levels are low in patients with Cushing's
disease[28], a pathological variety of hyperadrenocorticism.

People under high stress also release abnormal amounts of harmful adrenal steroids, resulting in glucose intolerance, athero-sclerosis, impaired immune function, cancer and brain disease. Melatonin may help slow these degenerative changes by damping pituitary/adrenal function.

The melatonin/corticoid relation has great significance since chronic hypercortisolemia has been linked with several aspects of aging. These include glucose intolerance (possibly leading to dia-betes), atherogenesis (leading to cardiovascular disease), impaired immune function, cancer[33] and age-related deterioration of the brain[34]. Furthermore, it is not only high absolute levels of corti-coids that are damaging, but disorganization of the normal rhythm of corticoid release. Corticoids are normally high in the early morning and daytime and low at night. Disorganized circadian cortisol rhythm (that is, loss of amplitude of the day/night pattern) and other phenomena indicative of dysfunctional pituitary/adre-nal function are characteristic of aging and have been described in subjects with senile dementia[34]. Properly timed melatonin intake may entrain (reorganize) this critical endocrine rhythm and lead to long-term systemic benefit. Indeed, the immune-enhancing and anti-corticoid effects of melatonin—or putative mediators of mela-tonin action—appear to depend on the nighttime administration of the melatonin[30, 35]. *Melatonin activity may represent an integral im-mune recovery mechanism: "the normal circadian release of melatonin may be seen as a kind of buffer device, quenching the adverse effects of stressful events on immune homeostasis"*[30].

Beta-receptor blockers ("beta-blockers"), which depress melato-nin secretion (see above), have immunosuppressive effects, but only when given in the evening[36]. This is when blood melatonin (and the immuno-enhancing effect of melatonin) is highest. Exoge-nous melatonin reverses beta-blocker-induced immunosuppression and enhances immune function in animals[36].

There is little literature on the use of melatonin in immunocom-promised states apart from cancer. A preliminary report on melatonin (20 mg/day in the evening) in AIDS patients revealed uneven, but generally beneficial effects on immune parameters[36]. Predictably, melatonin-induced corticoid antagonism and immune enhance-ment may not always be desirable. Melatonin exacerbated the pa-thology in one animal model of arthritis[37]. *Melatonin should be used cautiously, if at all, in autoimmune conditions and in cases of known or suspected adrenocortical insufficiency.*

MELATONIN VERSUS CANCER

It has been suggested that the steady increase in the incidence of cancer in the developed countries over the last 100 years is due to routine, artificial extension of the photoperiod by electric lights—"light pollution"[38]. A long photoperiod results in depressed melatonin during the night, when melatonin secretion should be high. The modern tendency to receive little exposure to natural lighting during much or most of the day may reduce the amplitude of the diurnal day/night cycle that is necessary for the proper production and secretion of melatonin. Remember, without some beta-receptor stimulation, which means bright light and activity during the day, melatonin secretion is lessened and the phases of secretion become confused. Whether or not "light pollution" is a factor in cancer epidemiology, there is an intriguing relation of the pineal gland and of melatonin to the development of malignancy, and supplementary melatonin may represent a new physiologic approach in cancer therapy.

Melatonin inhibits the incidence of chemically induced (DMBA) tumors in animals, which are increased by pineal suppression (long light phase) or pinealectomy[39]. Pinealectomy stimulates and/or melatonin inhibits the growth and sometimes the metastasis of experimental cancers of the lung, liver, ovary, pituitary and prostate and of melanoma and leukemia[40].

A persuasive hypothesis which was advanced nearly 20 years ago suggested that melatonin may play a key role in the prevention and even treatment of breast cancer[41]. Since then, substantial corroborative evidence has accumulated [39, 42]. For example, the circadian amplitude of melatonin was reduced by over half in patients with breast cancer versus patients with nonmalignant breast disease[43], and high urinary melatonin has been found in breast cancer patients in the morning[44], suggesting circadian disorganization. Melatonin downregulates estrogen receptors, inhibits estrogen-stimulated breast cancer growth and complements the oncostatic action of anti-estrogen drugs (tamoxifen)[45]. These actions have led to the suggestion that "melatonin may be the pineal gland's, and thus the body's own 'natural antiestrogen' "[45]. This may have implications for nonmalignant conditions associated with estrogen excess such as uterine fibroids, endometriosis and the premenstrual syndrome.

Melatonin may also have a special role in prostate and colorectal cancers. The circadian amplitude of melatonin is reduced by two-thirds in patients with prostate cancer versus patients with benign prostate disease, and a similar phenomenon was observed in colorectal cancer patients[43]. The possibility that the lower nocturnal melatonin levels were due to enhanced hepatic metabolism (destruction by the liver) rather than reduced secretion was ruled out by urinary metabolite analysis and suggests melatonin inadequacy in the dark period.

Melatonin can potentiate the action of immunostimulants given in cancer therapy. Melatonin (10-50 mg/day at 8 PM) potentiates interleukin-2 immunotherapy of pulmonary (lung) metastases[36]. Intramuscular melatonin (20 mg/day at 3 PM for two months, then 10 mg/day) given to 54 patients with metastatic solid tumors, mostly lung and colorectal, resulted in stabilized disease and improved quality of life for about 40 percent of the recipients[46].

Melatonin injections given in the morning stimulate tumor growth, in midafternoon have no effect and in the evening have a retarding effect[45,44]. This is consistent with the idea that the melatonin rhythm found in (tumor-free) youth and health is the one most conducive to those conditions.

MELATONIN, THE ANTI-AGING HORMONE?

The relation of age-related phenomena to melatonin loss and the case for melatonin as an anti-aging substance have been presented at length[11,34,75]. A representative of this hypothesis suggests that "the Melatonin Deficiency Syndrome is perhaps the basic mechanism through which aging changes can be explained in terms of a single causative lesion, a lesion that would cause the progressive patterns of change seen in the older population"[75]. Indeed, "the data accumulated to date certainly justify serious consideration of the possibility that supplemental melatonin may be beneficial during aging"[76].

Melatonin production declines with age in humans[77], and the nocturnal melatonin peak is almost completely lost[78]. This near-total loss of melatonin rhythmicity, because of the close reciprocal relation of melatonin and corticoids, is probably responsible for the pituitary/adrenal axis disinhibition that has been described as a characteristic of aging[34]. The adrenals of elderly humans are apparently hypersensitive to ACTH, and midnight corticoid levels (low in youth) are markedly elevated[79]. The effects of melatonin on both the release of corticoids and their peripheral effects, the pathogenic conditioning influence of corticoid excess and the phasic inhibitory influence of melatonin on the pituitary/adrenal axis were each discussed above. Modification of corticoid-related phenomena could explain much of melatonin's apparent anti-aging and other beneficial actions.

Blindness, which increases melatonin levels by virtue of effective constant darkness, or melatonin administration, both increase the life span of rats[76, 80]. Food restriction, a singularly effective anti-aging technique, upregulates melatonin synthesis while depressing most other endocrine functions[76]. This fact has led to the suggestion that the efficacy of food restriction derives from its effects on the pineal.

Melatonin can induce slow-wave sleep[75], which is a deeply restful type of sleep during which restoration of damaged tissue takes place. Slow-wave sleep declines with age. It has also been suggested that melatonin stimulates DNA repair mechanisms[75] and has indirect antioxidant activity by increasing cGMP (cyclic guanosine monophosphate) levels[34]. Neurochemical and neuropsychological features of dementia resemble some effects of melatonin deficiency, and nightly supplementary melatonin has been suggested for prevention of senile dementia[81].

Melatonin may have potential for long-term retarding of aging. In young, healthy individuals, reaction to the classic environmental cue (light/dark cycle) is robust and sufficient to produce a high-amplitude circadian pattern of melatonin levels. This in turn modulates many cyclic functions, especially the activity of the pituitary/adrenal axis. This allows the organism to recover from the day's (high-corticoid) stresses. With age, the body's endogenous melatonin declines, especially the nighttime peaks. Exogenous melatonin given in the late evening or before bed might act as chronobiotic replacement therapy by depressing cortisol release and by acting at precisely the time that cortisol levels should be lowest. This simulates the high-amplitude rhythm characteristic of youth—with all that implies.

This hypothesis finds some support in observations of tumor-bearing animals given melatonin as an experimental oncostatic (anti-tumor agent): "To our surprise chronic, circadian, night administration of melatonin resulted in a progressive, striking improvement of the general state of the mice and, most important, in a remarkable prolongation of life . . . astonishing differences in the fur and in the general condition of the [melatonin vs. control] groups (vigor, activity, posture) became increasingly evident"[26].

Melatonin is a powerful antioxidant; along with other antioxidants it could help prevent the cumulative free radical pathology associated with aging. In fact, a combination of melatonin, vitamins and accessory factors may have a significant impact on recovery from stress, immune function and age-related changes throughout the body. Some of the points have already been covered, but they will be reviewed here briefly within an antioxidant context.

The significance of the modulation of the pituitary/adrenal axis and modification of peripheral corticoid effects by melatonin, primarily through reduction of corticoids, is great since chronic hypercortisolemia has been linked with glucose intolerance, atherogenesis, impaired immune function and cancer[33]—all more or less aspects of the aging process. Excessive corticoid production is one aspect of overreaction to stress. However, one caveat is in order here regarding melatonin's positive effects: melatonin also increases growth hormone (GH) spikes[101], and excessive or inappropriate release of growth hormone is associated with incipient diabetes.

Co-administered nutrients may also play a role in modifying corticoid release and/or action on target tissues. There is a large mass of evidence indicating the possibility of blockading peripheral corticoid effects with pyridoxine derivatives[118]. These effects are mediated by the active pyridoxine metabolite pyridoxal-5-phosphate (P5P): P5P alters the binding of corticoids to nuclear receptors, thus modulating the hormone's actions. Deficiency of the vitamin, in contrast, enhances corticoid responsiveness[119]. In light of the positive mutual interaction of pyridoxine and melatonin, it would seem that pyridoxine/melatonin co-administration may optimize the effects of both on corticoid-related (stress) phenomena. Again, the marked synergy of riboflavin with pyridoxine calls for additional riboflavin, as well.

Vitamin A inhibits some peripheral effects of corticoids such as the depression of collagen synthesis[120] and of cell-mediated immunity[121]. Supplementary vitamin A ameliorates the impaired wound-healing, adrenal enlargement and (probably consequent) thymic and lymphoid suppression in experimental diabetes[122]. Because vitamin A is a fat-soluble vitamin with a potential for toxicity, care must be used, nevertheless, to avoid excessive dosages.

Zinc may modulate corticoid metabolism or action. Zinc-deficient animals have elevated levels of corticoids and associated defects of cell-mediated immunity[113, 123], and most of the behavioral effects of zinc deficiency in animals parallel the effects of corticoid and catecholamine excess[113]. Corticoids themselves induce zinc wasting[124], which suggests a vicious cycle of zinc depletion-induced stress and stress-induced zinc depletion. Supplementary zinc with pyridoxine reduces the excretion of catecholamine metabolites[125]— suggesting a general sedative and anti-stress effect. Zinc promotes vitamin A nutrition by enhancing the formation of the vitamin A-binding proteins which are needed to maintain normal blood levels of vitamin A. Zinc also acts as a membrane stabilizer[126] and renders cell membranes more resistant to toxic insults and oxidative damage[127]. Zinc itself contributes indirect antioxidant activity[128]. Because of its role in tissue healing, protein synthesis and oxidative stress protection, it has been suggested that zinc deficiency may be an important factor in aging[129].

The action of the B-complex vitamin niacinamide on cellular integrity in the face of oxidative injury may complement melatonin's prevention of oxidation-induced structural damage to DNA. Oxidative damage causes depletion of cellular NAD (nicotinamide adenine dinucleotide) which is used in the process of DNA repair[130]. Since NAD is also required for radical scavenging, NAD depletion has adverse effects on both processes. White blood cells are particularly sensitive to this depletion. However, supplementary niacinamide slows or stops NAD depletion.

Other actions of niacinamide tend to complement those of melatonin. Large doses of the vitamin—which are not recommended—have been used to reverse some parameters of age-related dysfunction.

Multigram doses (1-4 grams/day) produced marked enhancement of joint mobility, muscular strength, exercise tolerance and mood in a large human population[131]. These changes may well have been due to the indirect antioxidant effect of niacinamide and elevation by the vitamin of cellular NAD levels required for DNA repair. Large doses of niacinamide also have sedative, hypnotic, anticonvulsant, antiaggressive and muscle-relaxant activities in both animals and humans[132, 133]. These actions complement the sedative and hypnotic effects of melatonin.

Again, however, care must be exercised in the use of vitamin B-3. Gram dosages of this vitamin should only be used under medical supervision inasmuch as these amounts can cause liver damage, high levels of uric acid, unwanted skin pigmentation and diabetes.

OF SPECIAL INTEREST TO WOMEN

The potential role of melatonin in preventing/treating breast cancer was discussed above. In fact, melatonin has numerous actions which are consistent with both a preventive and a therapeutic role in breast cancer, particularly estrogen-sensitive types. Chronic use of high physiologic doses of melatonin (that is, 2 to 5 mg nightly) might be considered for long-term breast (and other) cancer prevention in high-risk women, keeping in mind, of course, that there may be other, as yet unknown, risks associated with this usage regimen. And if indeed melatonin is "the pineal gland's, and thus the body's own 'natural antiestrogen' "[45], then a variety of nonmalignant conditions associated with estrogen excess or estrogen/progesterone imbalance such as uterine fibroids, endometriosis and the premenstrual syndrome might also be ameliorated with melatonin. Melatonin appears to oppose the effects of excess estrogen while promoting the production of progesterone, which must be kept in balance with estrogen.

Recently, an hypothesis has been developed that melatonin might be involved in the prevention of osteoporosis[152] as follows:

- The incidence of osteoporosis increases with the age-related decline of melatonin levels.
- Melatonin can modulate the secretion of both calcitonin and parathyroid hormone—the hormones responsible for normal calcium metabolism and bone formation.
- Melatonin downregulates the pituitary/adrenal axis, which becomes disinhibited during aging; adrenal steroids are well-known inducers of bone loss.
- Immobility induces mobilization (loss) of bone minerals; immobility reduces plasma melatonin levels in animals; and exercise (a well-known positive affector of bone integrity) elevates melatonin levels in humans.
- Estrogens, which are already a mainstay in osteoporosis prevention and treatment, are known to elevate blood melatonin levels.

This hypothesis lacks empirical verification in the form of human clinical trials of melatonin in osteoporosis. Further, the antiestrogenic effects of melatonin would appear inconsistent with the hypothesis unless the therapeutic value of estrogen in osteoporosis is indeed a derivative of its effect on melatonin levels. Nevertheless, the case is sufficiently strong to warrant consideration of melatonin as an experimental adjunct in prevention and treatment—subordinate to the better-documented approaches (exercise, supplementation with calcium and magnesium and so on).

Another hypothesis holds that melatonin may be useful in the treatment and prevention of spontaneous abortion[105]. The key elements of this hypothesis are:

- Melatonin levels normally increase by 200 to 300 percent during the first two trimesters of pregnancy and fall abruptly at parturition.
- Melatonin decreases uterine contractility and stimulates the synthesis of progesterone, which also decreases uterine contractility.
- Progesterone may prevent immune-mediated embryo rejection.
- Pinealectomy increases the number of spontaneous abortions in animals.

If melatonin is used in women at risk of spontaneous abortion, the caution regarding melatonin in pregnancy should be observed.

Yet another hypothesis suggests that melatonin may help prevent endometrial hyperplasia (premalignancy) and cancer[153]. Facts favoring this hypothesis include:

- Melatonin has antiestrogenic actions and promotes the production of progesterone, an antiestrogen (estrogens increase the risk of hyperplasia and cancer).
- There are seasonal changes in the incidence of (premalignant) endometrial hyperplasia and anovulation, possibly associated with changes in melatonin levels.
- There is an increased incidence of endometrial hyperplasia after menopause and in obesity and diabetes—all of which are associated with rhythm disturbances and pineal dysfunction.

This hypothesis, too, lacks empirical verification, but provides a glimpse at future possibilities for clinical research with melatonin and its potential benefits to women. The possible significance of increased progesterone synthesis by melatonin[105, 154, 155] goes well beyond the scope of this book. Progesterone represents a very promising (if not proven) agent in the treatment of the premenstrual syndrome (PMS) and possibly other OB/GYN problems[156], including postpartum depression and psychosis.

Those considering using melatonin for treatment of PMS should read again the sections above which discuss the important role of exposure to light and high levels of activity during the day to increase the body's own production of melatonin.

One final note: At present melatonin is being researched as a major component in a contraceptive product. Quite large amounts of melatonin are required for this purpose, but women using melatonin should be aware that very elevated dosages of melatonin may influence fertility (see section "Safety and Potential Side Effects" below).

COMPLEMENTARY NUTRIENTS

Melatonin increases the formation of active pyridoxine (vitamin B-6) derivatives, which is vital to the vitamin's functions. The active pyridoxine metabolite pyridoxal-5-phosphate (P5P), which is a cofactor for many enzymes including the decarboxylases that are involved in the biosynthesis of serotonin and GABA, is formed by the action of pyridoxal kinase. Brain serotonin concentrations are increased by melatonin administration, and this has been attributed to its ability to stimulate the activity of brain pyridoxal kinase[61]. Another possibility is a sparing effect upon endogenous serotonin through supply of melatonin from an external source.

Pineal melatonin and serotonin levels are reduced in pyridoxine-deficient animals[107]. Pyridoxine deficiency also induces a marked (55 percent) reduction in serum melatonin at night along with a slight increase in the day, with the result that the night:day ratio decreases from 6:1 to about 2:1. Pineal melatonin levels are affected similarly, the night:day ratio decreasing from 46:1 to 19:1[107]. Thus, pyridoxine deficiency reduces not only total nighttime levels of melatonin, but dramatically reduces the amplitude of the circadian melatonin rhythm. (As noted above, robust amplitude, the dramatic nighttime production of melatonin in comparison with daytime production, may be more important than absolute levels of melatonin production and secretion.)

The pyridoxine/melatonin relationship is underscored by the clear effects of supplementary pyridoxine on relevant amino acid metabolism. The liver catabolizes the serotonin/melatonin precursor tryptophan via the enzyme tryptophan pyrrolase (TP; also known as tryptophan oxygenase). TP converts tryptophan into derivatives that are inactive as serotonin/melatonin precursors. Experimentally, large doses of pyridoxine (10 mg/kg, equivalent to about 600 to 800 mg in humans) reduces urinary excretion of TP products (suggesting enzyme inhibition) while increasing brain tryptophan, brain uptake of supplemental tryptophan and brain serotonin synthesis[108]. Much smaller doses of pyridoxine (0.5 mg/kg, about 30 to 40 mg) reduce the rise in urinary TP products in humans given moderately large tryptophan loads[109], indicating modification of TP activity at near-physiologic levels of pyridoxine intake.

It is possible that some of the reported neuropsychiatric benefits of supplementation with tryptophan[67] and pyridoxine[110] are due to melatonin enhancement. This idea has, in fact, been discussed at some length[26,111].

Melatonin restores numerous parameters of immunologic senescence in a way that precisely mirrors the action of zinc on the same parameters[112]. Melatonin can upregulate plasma zinc levels and normalizes zinc balance in senescent animals. Melatonin down regulates the adrenal steroids; the adrenal steroids, in turn, cause zinc wasting. Zinc deficiency augments adrenal steroid production and release, and adrenal steroids can depress melatonin secretion. Thus there is a multilateral and mutually reinforcing interrelation of zinc, melatonin and corticoids, with far-reaching implications for immunity, tissue healing, glucose tolerance, cardiovascular risk factors and aging in general. Further, pyridoxine greatly enhances zinc absorption[113], blocks peripheral corticoid actions and may enhance melatonin synthesis. All this suggests a mutual complementarity of melatonin, pyridoxine and zinc in immunologic, neuropsychiatric and metabolic applications and in general prevention of age-related deterioration.

It is germane to add detail here on pyridoxine forms for supplementary use. The active pyridoxine metabolite pyridoxal-5-phosphate (P5P) is in vogue in high-tech nutritional supplements, which appears at first to be a good idea: P5P would bypass pyridoxal kinase by supplying the preformed enzymic cofactor. Unfortunately, most P5P given orally is split by intestinal phosphatases into its constituents pyridoxal and phosphate[114, 115]. Further, only non-phosphorylated B-6 vitamers—not P5P itself—are taken up by the brain[116] and are generally more able to cross membranes than is P5P[115]. In other words, even if P5P were absorbed intact, it would have to be reduced to non-phosphorylated forms before it would become available to the central nervous system (CNS) and to most other tissues in the body. P5P is also very expensive. A simple and cheap form of pyridoxine (for example, HCl) co-administered with melatonin would be more cost-effective as well as useful for a broader range of effects. Lastly, additional coadministration of riboflavin may be advisable since P5P synthesis depends on this vitamin[117].

GETTING THE MOST FROM MELATONIN: DOSAGE AND TIMING

Fat-soluble substances are generally well-absorbed across oral and other mucous membranes; melatonin is fat-soluble. Orally administered melatonin in either regular or slow-release forms is absorbed readily and causes rapid serum melatonin increments with a high plateau for one to four hours thereafter[100]. Nasal delivery of melatonin may be more effective than the oral route, judging from the results of one trial in which small doses (1.7 mg) were used in this manner[20]. The authors of this study speculated that "the short way between the nasal cavities and the brain" might explain the high efficacy of such low doses, though avoidance of the high first-pass hepatic metabolism (destruction in the liver) and achievement of higher plasma levels of oral melatonin must also be factors. Sublingual lozenges and buccal patches mimic the effects of sprays. Melatonin taken with food appears to produce higher and steadier plasma levels than melatonin ingested during fasting.

The importance of circadian, nighttime administration of melatonin has been emphasized throughout. A dosing schedule after about 5 PM reconstitutes immunity in animals[30], restores normal circadian patterns of pituitary and adrenal hormones, improves sleep quality and mood in the absence of a pineal[101], retards tumor growth[44, 45] and mimics the pattern that is associated with neuropsychiatric normalcy and recovery from depression[50]. *Daytime melatonin administration may have opposite effects—disordered circadian rhythms, stimulated tumor growth, exacerbated depression, induced fatigue, drowsiness and slowed reaction time—and is to be avoided.*

Low-dose oral melatonin given at the appropriate times can produce marked changes in the settings of the internal clocks. For example, 2 mg of melatonin given to volunteers at 6 PM phase-advanced the circadian rhythm of (endogenous) melatonin, testosterone and probably corticoids[102], and *a minute dose (20 mcg) given by infusion over a 3-hour period starting at 4 PM or 8 PM likewise markedly phase-advanced the melatonin circadian rhythm*[103]. This means that quite small amounts of melatonin taken in a form which is not quickly destroyed by the liver and taken at an appropriate time can advance the internal cycles of the body by several hours.

Slow-release melatonin preparations have the advantage of elevating plasma melatonin concentrations for at least twice as long as ordinary oral tablets—about 5 to 7 hours. For individuals who have early morning insomnia, slow-release products will maintain high melatonin levels throughout the sleep period.

The use of melatonin in potentially sensitive special populations such as children and pregnant women warrants comment. The clinical experience with melatonin in children is slim, but available reports indicate positive effects in sleep disorders (along with an array of other benefits; see discussion above) with no side effects[24]. Caution might be advisable in children with delayed sexual development on account of the possible antigonadotropic effects of melatonin. There appears not to be any information on the teratogenicity of melatonin, or on the use of melatonin in pregnant women or in infants. Plasma melatonin levels normally increase by 200 to 300 percent during the first two trimesters[105], melatonin is present in human milk,[3] and prepubescent youth generally have higher levels of melatonin than adults. Melatonin levels decline toward the end of pregnancy, and in neonates melatonin levels are low for the first 3 months. It has been suggested that the precipitous drop in melatonin levels at parturition may dispose to postpartum depression and psychosis[106]. Caution suggests that melatonin should not be used during pregnancy or with young children or that it should be used only in minute amounts.

For further details on dose, see "Finding Your Optimal Personal Dose" in the Introduction.

SAFETY AND POTENTIAL SIDE EFFECTS

The acute toxicity of melatonin is extremely low. In animals an LD50 (lethal dose for 50 percent of the subjects) could not be established. Even 800 milligrams per kilogram bodyweight—a fantastically high dose—was not lethal[82]. Five human subjects were each given 1 gram per day for 25 to 30 days and were followed with an elaborate battery of physiologic and biochemical tests to detect potential toxicity; all findings were normal at the end of the test period[83]. Four subjects suffering from Parkinsonism were each given 1 gram daily for four weeks with "transitory sedation the only adverse reaction"[84]. One subject was given 200 mg intravenously daily for five days with no immediate or delayed toxicity even when reexamined 18 years later, and many investigators have used doses of 100 mg to 1.2 grams daily for days or weeks with few or no side effects[85].

In what must be some sort of record for extreme megadosing, 3.0 to 6.6 grams (3,000 to 6,600 mg)—the equivalent of over 1,300 5-mg tablets!—were given to 11 humans daily for 35 days without harm beyond isolated incidents of flushing, abdominal cramps, diarrhea and headaches[86], though the researchers noted that the subjects "reacted placidly" to these unpleasantries. This study was performed under USFDA auspices and was published in the *Journal of the American Medical Association*.

On account of its physiological actions there are a number of conditions and situations in which melatonin, given chronically, may have undesirable effects. These are largely theoretical concerns with little empirical verification at this time, but since recorded human experience with chronic supplementary melatonin is very limited, it is wise to be circumspect and aware of potential problems. After all, human populations which live close to the Arctic Circle—the Finnish, for example—have a record of depression which may well be tied to the amplitude of melatonin secretion during the Arctic winter. Other similarly geographically situated groups are noted for small but significant increases in the incidence of depression and/or manic/depressive mood disorders. Likewise, *the available published studies do not add up to a consistent picture of the more subtle effects of chronic melatonin use.* This point will be discussed below.

Animal studies suggest that melatonin can downregulate the pituitary/gonad axis resulting in hypogonadism (pathologically lessened sexual functioning or depressed activity of male sexual hormonal activity) and/or delayed puberty. (No human case of this has been reported.) However, though melatonin influences the timing of puberty in photoperiodic animals (animals that have seasonal cycles of reproduction) such as sheep, it does so marginally if at all in humans and nonphotoperiodic animals[1]. Nevertheless, the likelihood that humans may, in fact, be photoperiodic to some degree is suggested by melatonin's successful use as a contraceptive, which is discussed below. Chronic administration of low-dose melatonin in men did not alter blood levels of testosterone or luteinizing hormone[87]. Conflicting findings were presented in a recent review article on pediatric aspects of melatonin, and the author, in discussing potential therapeutic applications of melatonin, felt no need to mention delayed puberty as a potential side effect[88]. One case has been reported of extremely high melatonin levels associated with delayed puberty and hypogonadism[89]. Pubertal development and resolution of the hypogonadism occurred spontaneously as melatonin levels declined over several years. In this case, daytime melatonin levels exceeded normal by 15 to 20 times. It is thus possible that continuous (24-hour), very high melatonin levels could, over a period of many months or years, influence human pituitary/gonad activity and pubertal development, though a causal relationship is unclear.

There is preliminary work, on animals, which suggests that melatonin may accelerate the development of autoimmune conditions[37, 90]. One animal study indicated that melatonin given in large doses worsened collagen-induced arthritis, and there is (theoretical) reason to believe that melatonin may be harmful in autoimmune conditions such as multiple sclerosis. Melatonin has also transiently exacerbated neurological symptoms in one human multiple sclerosis (MS) sufferer[91], and a theoretical case has been made for the involvement of melatonin and pineal function in the development of MS[92]. One of the authors spoke with a woman for whom melatonin apparently caused symptomatic exacerbation of (preexisting)

Sjögren's syndrome, an unusual autoimmune condition. The symptoms abated after she stopped taking melatonin. The autoimmunity concern, like the hypogonadism concern, is still largely speculative. However, *supplementary melatonin should be used with caution, or not at all, in autoimmune conditions and chronic inflammatory conditions with a known or suspected autoimmune component,* until more and better information is available (see list of autoimmune conditions in the Appendix).

That melatonin may be undesirable for people with autoimmune conditions is consistent with the clearly documented action of melatonin as an immune enhancer[30] and corticoid antagonist[31]. On this basis it is possible that melatonin could have undesirable effects in chronic fatigue syndrome, in which pituitary/adrenal insufficiency has been documented[93], and melatonin would obviously have to be handled very cautiously in Addison's disease or milder forms of hypoadrenia. Again, these concerns are theoretical (no one has yet reported exacerbation of hypoadrenia with melatonin), but users beware.

Melatonin has been suggested for use as a contraceptive for women[94], which might raise the question of whether melatonin damages the female reproductive system. It does not. As a contraceptive, melatonin is used in very large doses (75 mg nightly) in a time-release form, so as to elevate blood levels drastically for a long period during the night. This usage effects changes in hypothalamic function which transiently oppose fertility. The reproductive system is fully functional and unharmed after melatonin is stopped. Notably, no side effects were evident in a contraception study giving women 300 mg of melatonin nightly for four months[95], and preliminary information from a recently completed Phase II clinical trial, in which 1,400 women were treated with 75 mg of melatonin nightly for four years, indicates that no side effects occurred other than the desired contraception[96].

As stated above, the safety of supplementary melatonin in pregnant and nursing women and for infants has not been studied. Melatonin has been used successfully (and without harm) to treat sleep disorders in children.

Melatonin has apparently precipitated reactions such as headache, insomnia, skin rash, upset stomach, nightmares and so on, but, as noted above, there is seemingly very poor consistency in the literature on the issue of side effects. However, they do appear to be dose-dependent. One author who is a practicing medical doctor found that out of 200 respondents to his survey, those taking 6 mg or more of melatonin per day commonly reported grogginess or lethargy for an hour or more in the morning. His figures indicate that perhaps 20 percent of those using melatonin at this 6 mg or more per day level suffered side effects[157]. Reduction of the dosage to 1 mg or less eliminated the side effects. This picture of the relation of melatonin intake to side effects is consistent with what we know of human populations exposed to dramatically varying amounts of sunlight. Frankly, the finding that humans can take 75 mg or even 300 mg melatonin per day without side effects of some sort, at the very least grogginess, does not appear reasonable unless the researchers conducting these "side effect-free" clinical trials were not looking for more subtle changes in mood and performance.

The likelihood of untoward effects on account of poor timing should be reemphasized. Although melatonin is indeed an exciting new adjunctive agent in the treatment of cancer and immune deficiency, poorly timed administration can have effects opposite of those desired. Melatonin injections given in the morning stimulate tumor growth [44, 45], while the same doses in midafternoon have no effect and in the evening have a retarding effect. And although some people with depression may suffer from a "low melatonin syndrome"[29], *any melatonin administration which unduly prolongs the nocturnal melatonin rise or which is given throughout the day may exacerbate Seasonal Affective Disorder*[73] *and bipolar and classic depression*[74]. Therefore, caution is indicated in all cases of depression, mania or mood disorders. As a practical matter, these effects are unlikely since consumers do not take "sleeping" pills in the daytime, but those who take enough melatonin to induce morning grogginess should consider cutting back.

Finally, animal studies have shown that moderately large doses of melatonin (equivalent in one study to about 30 mg in adult humans) increased light-induced damage to retinal photoreceptors[97]. The implication of this for individuals using commonly available commercial preparations (3 to 5 mg) is unknown. Further, in subjects given 250 mg of melatonin four times daily for 4 weeks, a battery of visual function tests revealed no evidence of retinal damage[83]. Our data on this point is inconsistent. Melatonin actually inhibits the proliferation of melanoma cells and the melanin synthesis in them[98], and melatonin is being tested as a treatment for malignant melanoma[99], a disease which is clearly linked to solar radiation. With respect to light exposure, then, melatonin may have protective effects as well. Still, it appears that the hormone may act as a mild photosensitizer (like chlorophyll or hypericin found in St. John's wort), at least for the eyes. Melatonin should be used cautiously when and if a great deal of bright light exposure is anticipated.

INCREASING *YOUR* BODY'S MELATONIN PRODUCTION

Three simple facts underlie any advice on increasing your body's melatonin production. First, remember that melatonin is released as part of a day/night or light/darkness cycle. Darkness and relative coolness increase melatonin production and the amplitude of melatonin levels in comparison with those found during the day. The reverse, bright light, especially bright light early in the day, inhibits the production of melatonin. Second, recall that melatonin production depends on prior stimulation of beta-receptors found on the surface of the pineal gland. Third, it is not the total or absolute amount of melatonin produced during the night, but the amplitude of the day/night rhythm (the magnitude of difference between nighttime production of melatonin and daytime suppression) that is most important for health.

These three facts mean that the body's production of melatonin depends on the difference between daytime and nighttime activity (or lack of activity). Practices which keep you wide awake during the day and which produce deep and restful sleep at night will increase melatonin production and the benefits of melatonin. Increase the "amplitude" of all your daily activities: make daytime more active and dynamic with plenty of light exposure and nighttime more passive and restful with low or no light.

Predictably, many suggestions (published by the authors elsewhere) regarding weight loss and general health maintenance apply here. The following short list constitutes a practical prescription in accord with the facts about melatonin production. Keep in mind the classic maxim: "sleep is not a luxury—it is a necessity."

1. Get more light early in the day. "Sleeping in" can blur the distinction between day and night and reduce the amplitude of

the associated cycles. (A currently popular light therapy technique, used in the treatment of some forms of depression, calls for bright light in the *early morning*, which probably enhances rhythm amplitude.)

2. Be physically active early in the day and limit naps to no more than 30 minutes. Physical activity turns off melatonin production during the day and raises the body's internal temperature. Daytime naps reverse this effect. If you nap, do so in the early or midafternoon (about 12 hours after the deepest sleep), which research has shown is the optimal time for napping.

3. Take a 30-minute walk either before or after breakfast or at your morning break. If you exercise, try to take your workouts in the morning rather than the evening. The pineal gland is like a clock which needs to be reset every day. Combining bright light and physical exertion is the most effective way to reset this clock. Outside light is generally brighter and of a fuller spectrum than inside light; it is better for you!

4. Avoid caffeine after the late afternoon and limit alcohol consumption in the evening. However, a cup of tea taken with supper helps some people sleep because a compound in tea opens up the circulation on the surface of the body and thus helps to lower the core temperature in preparation for sleep.

5. Eat larger and high-protein meals in the day, smaller and carbohydrate meals at night. Carbohydrates promote the delivery of tryptophan to the brain, and tryptophan is the raw material from which melatonin and serotonin are made. Carbohydrates are more conducive to sleep than are proteins.

6. Eat your last meal several hours before bedtime. Digestion temporarily raises the core temperature of the body, which is undesirable at bedtime. Too much food on the stomach also tends to interfere with early sleep and makes it difficult to awaken fully in the morning.

7. Avoid hard mental or physical work after about 6 PM. The secretion of stress hormones (adrenal cortical hormones) induced by hard work interferes with the production of serotonin and melatonin.

APPENDIX: AUTOIMMUNE CONDITIONS

Addison's disease
autoimmune gastritis
autoimmune myocarditis
autoimmune thyroiditis
(Hashimoto's)
autoimmune vasculitis
chronic fibrositis
dermatomyositis
fibromyalgia
hepatitis
hypopigmentation (vitiligo)
idiopathic thrombocytopenia
interstitial cystitis (Hunner's
ulcer)

Klinefelter's syndrome
(hypogonadism)
lupus erythematosus
multiple sclerosis
myasthenia gravis
nephritis
osteomyelitis
ovaritis
pernicious anemia
polymyositis
progressive systemic sclerosis
(scleroderma)
rheumatoid arthritis
Sjögren's syndrome
Type I diabetes mellitus
ulcerative colitis

References

1. Clin Endocrinol 29: 205-29, 1988.
2. NY Acad Sci Ann 719: 146-58, 1994.
3. J Clin Endocrinol Metab 77: 838-41, 1993.
4. J Pineal Res 18: 28-31, 1995.
5. Biochem Mol Bio Int 35: 627-34, 1995.
6. Biol Psychiatry 23: 405-25, 1988.
7. Life Sci 23: 2257-74, 1978.
8. Am J Psychiatry 145: 52-6, 1988.
9. Lancet ii: 1235-37, 1974.

10. Psychopharmacology **97**: 285-94, 1989.
11. Med Hypotheses **34**: 300-9, 1991.
12. J Neural Transm Suppl 21: 233-41, 1986.
13. Br Med J **298**: 705-7, 1989.
14. Biol Psychiatry **33**: 526-30, 1993.
15. Lancet **337**: 1121-4, 1991.
16. J Neurol Neurosurg Psychiatry **55**: 665-70, 1992.
17. Peptides **1**: 281-4, 1980.
18. Psychopharmacology **100**: 222-6, 1990.
19. NY Acad Sci Ann **453**: 242-52, 1985.
20. Adv Biosci **29**: 327-9, 1981.
21. Neurosci Lett **45**: 317-21, 1984.
22. Proc Natl Acad Sci USA **91**: 1824-8, 1994.
23. N Engl J Med **328**: 1230-5, 1993.
24. Dev Med Child Neurol **36**: 97-107, 1994.
25. Int J Neurosci **52**: 239-40, 1990.
26. Med Hypotheses **31**: 233-42, 1990.
27. Neuroendocrinology **10**: 139-54, 1972.
28. Psychoneuroendocrinology **8**: 75-80, 1983.
29. Acta Psychiatr Scand **71**: 319-30, 1985.
30. J Neuroimmunol **13**: 19-30, 1986.
31. Jpn J Exp Med **54**: 255-61, 1984.
32. Brain Res **450**: 18-24, 1988.
33. Med Hypotheses **7**: 315-31, 1981.
34. Int J Neurosci **52**: 85-92, 1990.
35. Int J Immunopharmacol **11**: 333-40, 1989.
36. Melatonin and the Pineal Gland— From Basic Science to Clinical Application. Elsevier, New York, 1993, pages 295-302.
37. J Neuroimmunol **39**: 23-30, 1992.
38. Med Hypotheses **33**: 75-8, 1990.
39. Cancer Invest **5**: 379-85, 1987.
40. Role of Melatonin and Pineal Peptides in Neuroimmunomodulation. Plenum, New York, 1991, pages 243-51.
41. Lancet **ii**: 814-6, 1978.
42. Eur J Cancer Clin Oncol **28**: 501-3, 1992.
43. Melatonin and the Pineal Gland— From Basic Science to Clinical Application. Elsevier, New York, 1993, pages 311-6.
44. J Neural Transm **52**: 269-79, 1981.
45. Role of Melatonin and Pineal Peptides in Neuroimmunomodulation. Plenum, New York (NY), 1991, pages 233-40.
46. Oncology **48**: 448-50, 1991.
47. Psychoneuroendocrinology **9**: 261-77, 1984.
48. Int J Clin Pharmacol Res **9**: 159-64, 1989.
49. Am J Psychiatry **142**: 811-6, 1985.
50. Psychiatry Res **28**: 263-78, 1989.
51. Arch Gen Psychiatry **35**: 769-71, 1978.
52. Am J Psychiatry **146**: 829-39, 1989.
53. South Med J **77**: 1516-8, 1984.
54. Adv Biosci **29**: 197-9, 1981.
55. Adv Biol Psychiatry **10**: 176-99, 1983.
56. Adv Biol Psychiatry **10**: 148-59, 1983.
57. The Pharmacological Basis of Therapeutics. Macmillan, New York, 1980, pages 391-447.
58. Biol Psychiatry **21**: 406-10, 1986.
59. The Pharmacological Basis of Therapeutics. Macmillan, New York, 1980, pages 176-210.
60. Acta Med Scand **221**: 155-8, 1987.
61. The Pineal Gland. Churchill Livingstone, London, 1971, pages 213-27.
62. NY Acad Sci Ann **487**: 202-20, 1986.

63. NY Acad Sci Ann **487**: 150-67, 1986.
64. Behav Brain Sci **9**: 345-6, 1986.
65. Prog Neuropsychopharmacol Biol Psychiatry **11**: 173-77, 1987.
66. Biol Psychiatry **22**: 205-12, 1987.
67. Nutr Brain **7**: 49-88, 1986.
68. J Psychiatr Res **17**: 107-13, 1982/3.
69. Photodermatol **5**: 107-9, 1988.
70. Chronobiology and Psychiatric Disorders. Elsevier, New York, 1987, pages 181-206.
71. Psychopathology **19** (Suppl 2): 136-41, 1986.
72. Biol Psychiatry **33**: 54-7, 1993.
73. NY Acad Sci Ann **453**: 260-9, 1985.
74. Am J Psychiatry **133**: 1181-6, 1976.
75. Med Hypotheses **23**: 337-52, 1987.
76. BioEssays **14**: 169-75, 1992.
77. J Clin Endocrinol Metab **66**: 648-52, 1988.
78. J Clin Endocrinol Metab **55**: 27-9, 1982.
79. J Gerontol **24**: 292-7, 1969.
80. J Chronic Dis **34**: 427-8, 1981.
81. Med Hypotheses **24**: 59-68, 1987.
82. Nature **214**: 919-20, 1967.
83. J Clin Endocrinol Metab **45**: 768-74, 1977.
84. Lancet **i**: 271, 1973.
85. J Neural Transm Suppl 13: 339-47, 1978.
86. J Am Med Assoc **221**: 88, 1972.
87. Clin Endocrinol **24**: 375-82, 1986.
88. J Pediatr **123**: 843-51, 1993.
89. N Engl J Med **327**: 1356-9, 1992.
90. Autoimmunity **17**: 83-6, 1994.
91. Int J Neurosci **66**: 237-50, 1992.
92. Int J Neurosci **63**: 206-15, 1992.
93. J Clin Endocrinol Metab **73**: 1224-34, 1991.
94. Eur J Obstet Gynecol Reprod Biol **49**: 3-9, 1993.
95. J Clin Endocrinol Metab **74**: 108-17, 1992.

96. Ms. Jo Robinson, personal communication. (Presently collaborating with Russell Reiter on a book about melatonin.)
97. Invest Ophthalmol Visual Sci **33**: 1894-902, 1992.
98. Exp Cell Res **206**: 189-94, 1993.
99. Melanoma Res **1**: 237-43, 1991.
100. Neuroendocrinology **39**: 307-13, 1984.
101. Brain Res Bull **27**: 181-5, 1991.
102. J Pineal Res **9**: 113-24, 1990.
103. Melatonin and the Pineal Gland— From Basic Science to Clinical Application. Elsevier, New York, 1993, pages 235-9.
104. Eur J Clin Pharmacol **38**: 297-301, 1990.
105. Int J Neurosci **62**: 243-50, 1992.
106. Int J Neurosci **62**: 101-5, 1992.
107. Neurosci Biobehav Rev **12**: 189-93, 1988.
108. J Neurochem **43**: 733-6, 1984.
109. Br J Clin Pharmacol **10**: 617-9, 1980.
110. Biol Psychiatry **29**: 931-41, 1991.
111. Int J Neurosci **52**: 225-32, 1990.
112. NY Acad Sci Ann **719**: 298-307, 1994.
113. Biol Psychiatry **17**: 513-32, 1982.
114. Gastroenterology **91**: 343-50, 1986.
115. Vitamins. Walter de Gruyter, New York, 1988, pages 543-618.
116. Nutr Brain **3**: 265-99, 1979.
117. Physiol Rev **69**: 1170-97, 1989.
118. Endocr Rev **7**: 140-8, 1986.
119. NY Acad Sci Ann **585**: 452-65, 1990.
120. Ann Surg **177**: 222-7, 1973.
121. J Immunol **111**: 1376-82, 1973.
122. Ann Surg **194**: 42-50, 1981.
123. J Nutr **109**: 1847-55, 1979.
124. Lancet **ii**: 1169-72, 1971.
125. Excerpta Med—Psychiatry **42**: 70, 1980.

126. Med Clin North Am **60**: 799-812, 1976.
127. Life Sci **28**: 1425-38, 1981.
128. Lancet **i**: 191-2, 1978.
129. Med Hypotheses **19**: 117-37, 1986.
130. Drugs **42**: 569-605, 1991.
131. J Am Geriatr Soc **3**: 927-36, 1955.
132. Experientia **32**: 1036-7, 1976.
133. Nature **278**: 563-5, 1979.
134. The Neuropsychology of Sleep and Dreaming. Lawrence Erlbaum Associates, Hillsdale (NJ), 1992, pages 289-303.
135. Med Hypotheses **44**: 39-46, 1995.
136. Med Hypotheses **36**: 195-9, 1991.
137. Life Sci **10p1**: 841-50, 1971.
138. The Pharmacological Basis of Therapeutics. Macmillan, New York, 1980, pages 339-75.
139. Med Hypotheses **23**: 433-40, 1987.
140. South Med J **77**: 1491-3, 1984.
141. Mental and Elemental Nutrients. Keats, New Canaan (CT), 1975, pages 422-31.
142. Med Hypotheses **26**: 255-7, 1988.
143. Methods Find Exp Clin Pharmacol **10**: 243-5, 1988.
144. Life Extension: A Practical Scientific Approach. Warner, New York, 1982, page 195.
145. Sleep **13**: 15-23, 1990.
146. Experientia **48**: 716-20, 1992.
147. Trends Pharmacol Sci **9**: 278-9, 1988.
148. The Merck Index. Merck and Company, Rahway (NJ), 1989, pages 1272-3.
149. Med Hypotheses **19**: 185-98, 1986.
150. Fundam Clin Pharmacol **4**: 169-74, 1990.
151. Acta Psychiatr Belg **76**: 658-66, 1976.
152. Int J Neurosci **62**: 215-25, 1992.
153. Int J Neurosci **62**: 89-96, 1992.
154. J Endocrinol **119**: 523-30, 1988.
155. J Reprod Fertil **84**: 669-77, 1988.
156. The Premenstrual Syndrome and Progesterone Therapy. Year Book Medical Publishers, Inc, Chicago, 1984.
157. Melatonin: Nature's Sleeping Pill. Be Happier Press, Marina Del Rey (CA), 1995.